MW00508659

Slow Cooker Fish Recipes

The Best Collection Of Fish Recipes

By Wanda Gordon

Sommario

Introduction

We understand you are constantly seeking less complicated means to prepare your meals. We additionally recognize you are possibly sick and tired of investing long hours in the kitchen food preparation with numerous frying pans and pots.

Well, currently your search is over! We found the excellent cooking area device you can utilize from now on! We are talking about the Slow stove! These remarkable pots enable you to prepare a few of the best recipes ever with minimal effort

Slow cookers prepare your meals much easier and also a lot healthier! You don't require to be an expert in the kitchen area to prepare a few of the most tasty, flavorful, textured as well as rich recipes!

All you require is your Slow stove as well as the appropriate active ingredients! This fantastic recipe book you are about to discover will certainly teach you how to prepare the very best slow-moving prepared dishes.

It will certainly show you that you can make some impressive morning meals, lunch recipes, side meals, chicken, meat as well as fish recipes.

Lastly yet importantly, this recipe book supplies you some straightforward as well as pleasant desserts.

Slow Cooker Fish Recipes

Salmon and Green Onions Mix

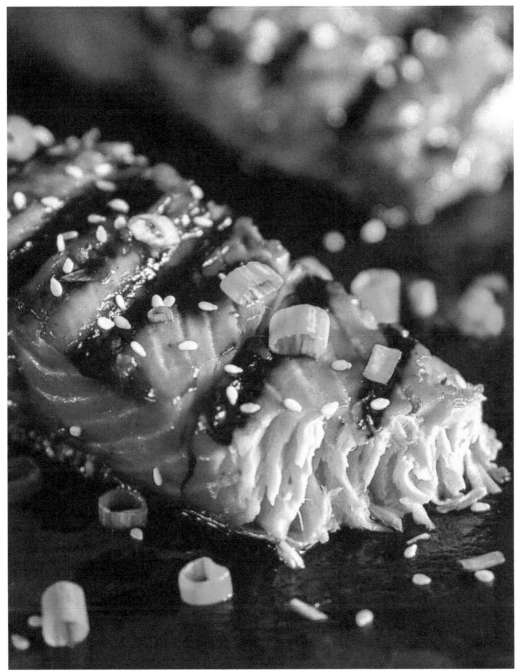

Preparation time: 10 minutes
Cooking time: 2 hours
Servings: 4

Ingredients:
- 1 green onions bunch, halved

- 10 tablespoons lemon juice
- 4 salmon fillets, boneless
- Salt and black pepper to the taste
- 2 tablespoons avocado oil

Directions:
1. Grease your Slow cooker with the oil, add salmon, top with onion, lemon juice, salt and pepper, cover, cook on High for 2 hours, divide everything between plates and serve.

Nutrition: calories 260, fat 3, fiber 1, carbs 14, protein 14

Shrimp Mix

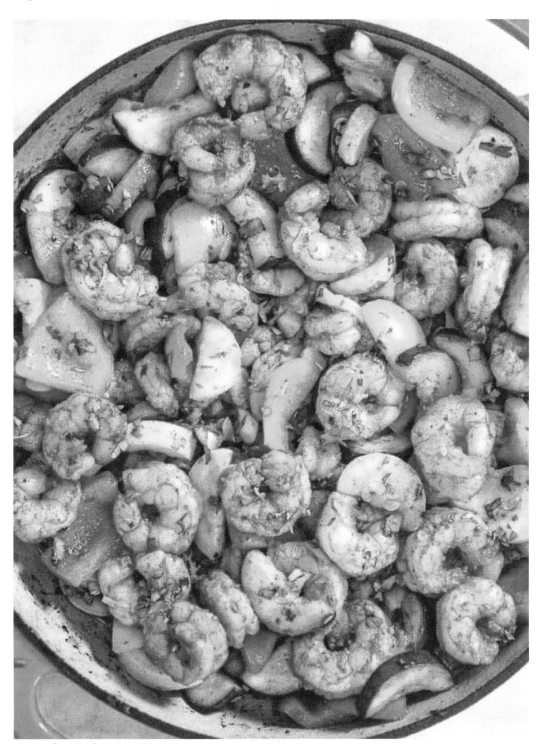

Preparation time: 10 minutes
Cooking time: 1 hour and 30 minutes
Servings: 4

Ingredients:

- 2 tablespoons olive oil
- 1 pound shrimp, peeled and deveined
- ¼ cup chicken stock
- 1 tablespoon garlic, minced
- 2 tablespoons parsley, chopped
- Juice of ½ lemon
- Salt and black pepper to the taste

Directions:
1. Put the oil in your Slow cooker, add stock, garlic, parsley, lemon juice, salt and pepper and whisk really well.
2. Add shrimp, stir, cover, cook on High for 1 hour and 30 minutes, divide into bowls and serve.

Nutrition: calories 240, fat 4, fiber 3, carbs 9, protein 3

Paprika Cod

Preparation time: 10 minutes
Cooking time: 3 hours
Servings: 2

Ingredients:
- 1 tablespoon olive oil
- 1 pound cod fillets, boneless
- 1 teaspoon sweet paprika
- ¼ cup chicken stock
- ¼ cup white wine
- 2 scallions, chopped
- ½ teaspoon rosemary, dried
- A pinch of salt and black pepper

Directions:
1. In your slow cooker, mix the cod with the paprika, oil and the other ingredients, toss gently, put the lid on and cook on High for 3 hours.
2. Divide everything between plates and serve.

Nutrition: calories 211, fat 8, fiber 4, carbs 8, protein 8

Asian Steamed Fish

Preparation time: 10 minutes
Cooking time: 1 hour
Servings: 4

Ingredients:
- 2 tablespoons sugar
- 4 salmon fillets, boneless
- 2 tablespoons soy sauce
- ¼ cup olive oil
- ¼ cup veggie stock
- 1 small ginger piece, grated
- 6 garlic cloves, minced
- 2 tablespoons Worcestershire sauce
- 1 bunch leeks, chopped
- 1 bunch cilantro, chopped

Directions:
1. Put the oil in your slow cooker, add leeks and top with the fish.
2. In a bowl, mix stock with ginger, sugar, garlic, cilantro and soy sauce, stir, add this over fish, cover and cook on High for 1 hour.
3. Divide fish between plates and serve with the sauce drizzled on top.

Nutrition: calories 300, fat 8, fiber 2, carbs 12, protein 6

Spicy Tuna

Preparation time: 10 minutes
Cooking time: 2 hours
Servings: 2

Ingredients:
- 1 pound tuna fillets, boneless and cubed
- ½ teaspoon red pepper flakes, crushed
- ¼ teaspoon cayenne pepper
- ½ cup chicken stock
- ½ teaspoon chili powder
- 1 tablespoon olive oil
- A pinch of salt and black pepper
- 1 tablespoon chives, chopped

Directions:
1. In your slow cooker, mix the tuna with the pepper flakes, cayenne and the other ingredients, toss, put the lid on and cook on High for 2 hours.
2. Divide the tuna mix between plates and serve.

Nutrition: calories 193, fat 7, fiber 3, carbs 6, protein 6

Poached Cod and Pineapple Mix

Preparation time: 10 minutes
Cooking time: 4 hours
Servings: 2

Ingredients:
- 1 pound cod, boneless
- 6 garlic cloves, minced
- 1 small ginger pieces, chopped
- ½ tablespoon black peppercorns
- 1 cup pineapple juice
- 1 cup pineapple, chopped
- ¼ cup white vinegar
- 4 jalapeno peppers, chopped
- Salt and black pepper to the taste

Directions:
1. Put the fish in your crock, season with salt and pepper.
2. Add garlic, ginger, peppercorns, pineapple juice, pineapple chunks, vinegar and jalapenos.
3. Stir gently, cover and cook on Low for 4 hours.
4. Divide fish between plates, top with the pineapple mix and serve.

Nutrition: calories 240, fat 4, fiber 4, carbs 14, protein 10

Ginger Tuna

Preparation time: 5 minutes
Cooking time: 2 hours
Servings: 2

Ingredients:
- 1 pound tuna fillets, boneless and roughly cubed
- 1 tablespoon ginger, grated
- 1 red onion, chopped
- 2 teaspoons olive oil
- Juice of 1 lime
- ¼ cup chicken stock
- 1 tablespoon chives, chopped
- A pinch of salt and black pepper

Directions:
1. In your slow cooker, mix the tuna with the ginger, onion and the other ingredients, toss, put the lid on and cook on High for 2 hours.
2. Divide the mix into bowls and serve.

Nutrition: calories 200, fat 11, fiber 4, carbs 5, protein 12

Chili Catfish

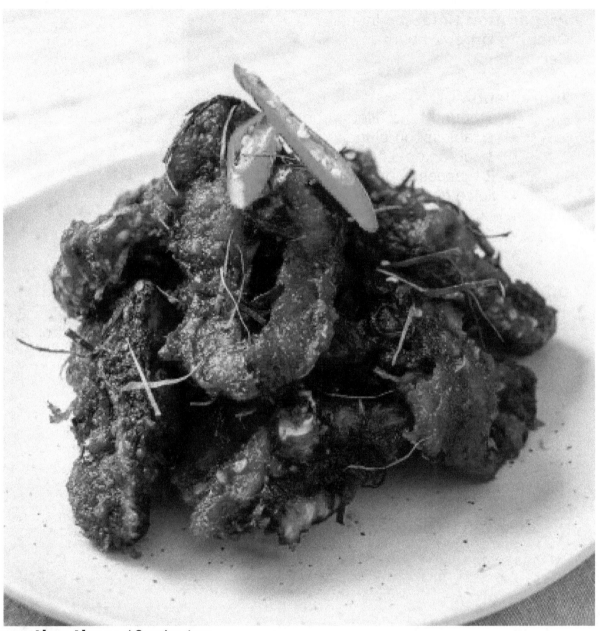

Preparation time: 10 minutes
Cooking time: 6 hours
Servings: 4

Ingredients:
- 1 catfish, boneless and cut into 4 pieces
- 3 red chili peppers, chopped
- ½ cup sugar
- ¼ cup water
- 1 tablespoon soy sauce

- 1 shallot, minced
- A small ginger piece, grated
- 1 tablespoon coriander, chopped

Directions:
1. Put catfish pieces in your Slow cooker.
2. Heat up a pan with the coconut sugar over medium-high heat and stir until it caramelizes.
3. Add soy sauce, shallot, ginger, water and chili pepper, stir, pour over the fish, add coriander, cover and cook on Low for 6 hours.
4. Divide fish between plates and serve with the sauce from the slow cooker drizzled on top.

Nutrition: calories 200, fat 4, fiber 4, carbs 8, protein 10

Chives Shrimp

Preparation time: 10 minutes
Cooking time: 1 hour
Servings: 2

Ingredients:
- 1 pound shrimp, peeled and deveined
- 1 tablespoon chives, chopped
- ½ teaspoon basil, dried
- 1 teaspoon turmeric powder
- 1 tablespoon olive oil
- ½ cup chicken stock

Directions:
1. In your slow cooker, mix the shrimp with the basil, chives and the other ingredients, toss, put the lid on and cook on High for 1 hour.
2. Divide the shrimp between plates and serve with a side salad.

Nutrition: calories 200, fat 12, fiber 3, carbs 7, protein 9

Tuna Loin Mix

Preparation time: 10 minutes
Cooking time: 4 hours and 10 minutes
Servings: 2

Ingredients:
- ½ pound tuna loin, cubed
- 1 garlic clove, minced
- 4 jalapeno peppers, chopped
- 1 cup olive oil
- 3 red chili peppers, chopped
- 2 teaspoons black peppercorns, ground
- Salt and black pepper to the taste

Directions:
1. Put the oil in your Slow cooker, add chili peppers, jalapenos, peppercorns, salt, pepper and garlic, whisk, cover and cook on Low for 4 hours.
2. Add tuna, stir again, cook on High for 10 minutes more, divide between plates and serve.

Nutrition: calories 200, fat 4, fiber 3, carbs 10, protein 4

Coriander Salmon Mix

Preparation time: 5 minutes
Cooking time: 3 hours
Servings: 2

Ingredients:
- 1 pound salmon fillets, boneless and roughly cubed
- 1 tablespoon coriander, chopped
- ½ teaspoon chili powder
- ¼ cup chicken stock
- 3 scallions, chopped
- Juice of 1 lime
- 2 teaspoons avocado oil
- A pinch of salt and black pepper

Directions:
1. In your slow cooker, mix the salmon with the coriander, chili powder and the other ingredients, toss gently, put the lid on and cook on High for 3 hours.
2. Divide the mix between plates and serve.

Nutrition: calories 232, fat 10, fiber 4, carbs 6, protein 9

Creamy Sea Bass

Preparation time: 10 minutes
Cooking time: 1 hour and 30 minutes
Servings: 2

Ingredients:
- 1 pound sea bass
- 2 scallion stalks, chopped
- 1 small ginger piece, grated
- 1 tablespoon soy sauce
- 2 cups coconut cream
- 4 bok choy stalks, chopped
- 3 jalapeno peppers, chopped
- Salt and black pepper to the taste

Directions:
1. Put the cream in your Slow cooker, add ginger, soy sauce, scallions, a pinch of salt, black pepper, jalapenos, stir, top with the fish and bok choy, cover and cook on High for 1 hour and 30 minutes.
2. Divide the fish mix between plates and serve.

Nutrition: calories 270, fat 3, fiber 3, carbs 18, protein 17

Tuna and Green Beans

Preparation time: 10 minutes
Cooking time: 3 hours
Servings: 2

Ingredients:
- 1 pound tuna fillets, boneless
- 1 cup green beans, trimmed and halved
- ½ cup chicken stock
- ½ teaspoon sweet paprika
- ½ teaspoon garam masala
- 3 scallions, minced
- ½ teaspoon ginger, ground
- 1 tablespoon olive oil
- 1 tablespoon chives, chopped
- Salt and black pepper to the taste

Directions:
1. In your slow cooker, mix the tuna with the green beans, stock and the other ingredients, toss gently, put the lid on and cook on High for 3 hours.
2. Divide the mix between plates and serve.

Nutrition: calories 182, fat 7, fiber 3, carbs 6, protein 9

Flavored Cod Fillets

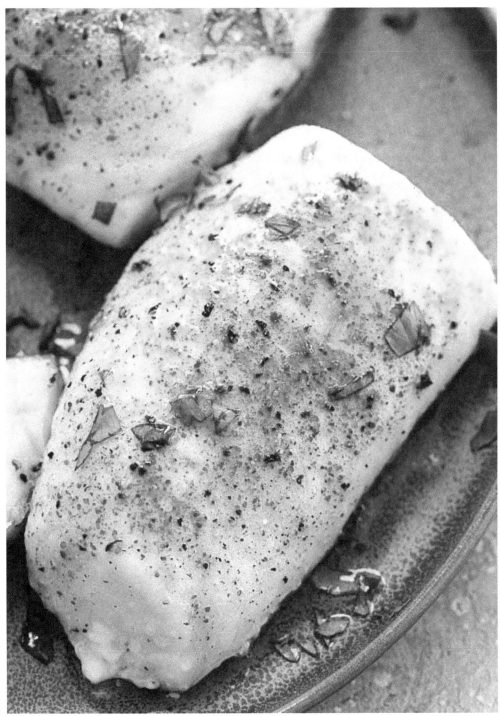

Preparation time: 10 minutes
Cooking time: 2 hours
Servings: 4

Ingredients:
- 4 medium cod fillets, boneless

- ¼ teaspoon nutmeg, ground
- 1 teaspoon ginger, grated
- Salt and black pepper to the taste
- 1 teaspoon onion powder
- ¼ teaspoon sweet paprika
- 1 teaspoon cayenne pepper
- ½ teaspoon cinnamon powder

Directions:
1. In a bowl, mix cod fillets with nutmeg, ginger, salt, pepper, onion powder, paprika , cayenne black pepper and cinnamon, toss, transfer to your Slow cooker, cover and cook on Low for 2 hours.
2. Divide between plates and serve with a side salad.

Nutrition: calories 200, fat 4, fiber 2, carbs 14, protein 4

Cod and Corn

Preparation time: 5 minutes
Cooking time: 2 hours
Servings: 2

Ingredients:
- 1 pound cod fillets, boneless
- 1 tablespoon avocado oil
- ½ teaspoon chili powder
- ½ teaspoon coriander, ground
- 1 cup corn
- ½ tablespoon lime juice
- 1 tablespoon chives, chopped
- ¼ cup chicken stock
- A pinch of salt and black pepper

Directions:
1. In your slow cooker, mix the cod with the oil, corn and the other ingredients, toss, put the lid on and cook on High for 2 hours.
2. Divide the mix between plates and serve.

Nutrition: calories 210, fat 8, fiber 3, carbs 6, protein 14

Shrimp and Baby Carrots Mix

Preparation time: 10 minutes
Cooking time: 4 hours and 30 minutes
Servings: 2

Ingredients:
- 1 small yellow onion, chopped
- 15 baby carrots
- 2 garlic cloves, minced
- 1 small green bell pepper, chopped
- 8 ounces canned coconut milk
- 3 tablespoons tomato paste
- ½ teaspoon red pepper, crushed
- ¾ tablespoons curry powder
- ¾ tablespoon tapioca flour
- 1 pound shrimp, peeled and deveined

Directions:
1. In your food processor, mix onion with garlic, bell pepper, tomato paste, coconut milk, red pepper and curry powder, blend well, add to your Slow cooker, also add baby carrots, stir, cover and cook on Low for 4 hours.
2. Add tapioca and shrimp, stir, cover and cook on Low for 30 minutes more.
3. Divide into bowls and serve.

Nutrition: calories 230, fat 4, fiber 3, carbs 14, protein 5

Turmeric Salmon

Preparation time: 5 minutes
Cooking time: 2 hours
Servings: 2

Ingredients:
- 1 pound salmon fillets, boneless
- 1 red onion, chopped
- ½ teaspoon turmeric powder
- ½ teaspoon oregano, dried
- ½ cup chicken stock
- 1 teaspoon olive oil
- Salt and black pepper to the taste
- 1 tablespoon chives, chopped

Directions:
1. In your slow cooker, mix the salmon with the turmeric, onion and the other ingredients, toss gently, put the lid on and cook on High for 2 hours.
2. Divide the mix between plates and serve.

Nutrition: calories 200, fat 12, fiber 3, carbs 6, protein 11

Dill Trout

Preparation time: 10 minutes
Cooking time: 2 hours
Servings: 4

Ingredients:
- 2 lemons, sliced
- ¼ cup chicken stock
- Salt and black pepper to the taste
- 2 tablespoons dill, chopped
- 12 ounces spinach
- 4 medium trout

Directions:
1. Put the stock in your Slow cooker, add the fish inside, season with salt and pepper, top with lemon slices, dill and spinach, cover and cook on High for 2 hours.
2. Divide fish, lemon and spinach between plates and drizzle some of the juice from the slow cooker all over.

Nutrition: calories 240, fat 5, fiber 4, carbs 9, protein 14

Sea Bass and Chickpeas

Preparation time: 5 minutes
Cooking time: 3 hours
Servings: 2

Ingredients:
- 1 pound sea bass fillets, boneless
- ½ cup chicken stock
- ½ cup canned chickpeas, drained and rinsed
- 2 tablespoons tomato paste
- ½ teaspoon rosemary, dried
- ½ teaspoon oregano, dried
- 2 scallions, minced
- 1 tablespoon olive oil
- Salt and black pepper to the taste

Directions:
1. In your slow cooker, mix the sea bass with the chickpeas, stock and the other ingredients, toss, put the lid on and cook on High for 3 hours.
2. Divide everything between plates and serve.

Nutrition: calories 132, fat 9, fiber 2, carbs 5, protein 11

Fish Pie

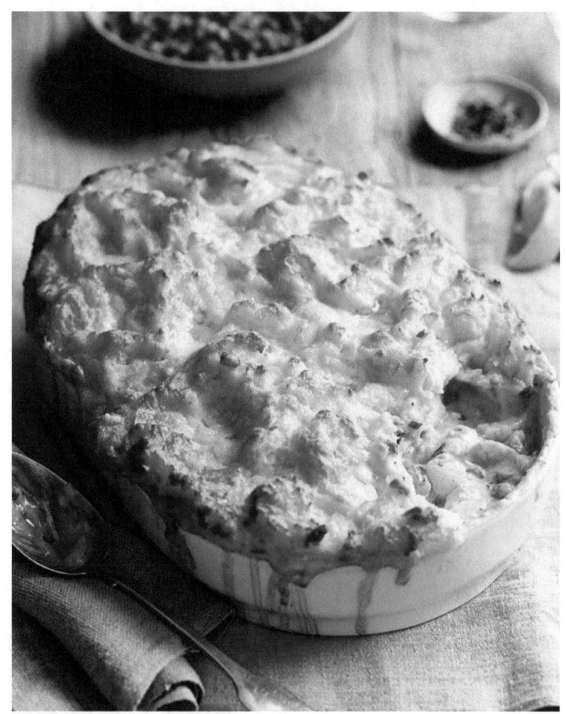

Preparation time: 10 minutes
Cooking time: 2 hours and 30 minutes
Servings: 6

Ingredients:
- 1 red onion, chopped

- 2 salmon fillets, skinless and cut into medium pieces
- 2 mackerel fillets, skinless and cut into medium pieces
- 3 haddock fillets and cut into medium pieces
- 2 bay leaves
- ¼ cup butter+ 2 tablespoons
- 1 cauliflower head, florets separated and riced
- 4 eggs, hard-boiled, peeled and sliced
- 4 cloves
- 1 cup whipping cream
- ½ cup water
- A pinch of nutmeg, ground
- 1 cup cheddar cheese, shredded+ ½ cup
- 1 tablespoon parsley, chopped
- Salt and black pepper to the taste
- 4 tablespoons chives, chopped

Directions:
1. Put cream and ½ cup water in your Slow cooker,, add salmon, mackerel and haddock, onion, cloves and bay leaves, cover and cook on High for 1 hour and 30 minutes
2. Add nutmeg, eggs, 1 cup cheese, ¼ cup butter, cauliflower rice, the rest of the cheddar, chives, parsley, salt, pepper and the rest of the butter, cover and cook on High for 1 more hour.
3. Slice pie, divide between plates and serve.

Nutrition: calories 300, fat 45, fiber 3, carbs 5, protein 26

Creamy Shrimp

Preparation time: 10 minutes
Cooking time: 1 hour
Servings: 2

Ingredients:
- 1 pound shrimp, peeled and deveined
- 2 scallions, chopped
- ¼ cup chicken stock
- 2 tablespoons avocado oil
- ½ cup heavy cream
- 1 teaspoon garam masala
- 1 tablespoon ginger, grated
- A pinch of salt and black pepper
- 1 tablespoon parsley, chopped

Directions:
1. In your slow cooker, mix the shrimp with the scallions, stock and the other ingredients, toss, put the lid on and cook on High for 1 hour.
2. Divide the mix into bowls and serve.

Nutrition: calories 200, fat 12, fiber 2, carbs 6, protein 11

Slow Cooked Haddock

Preparation time: 10 minutes
Cooking time: 2 hours
Servings: 4

Ingredients:
- 1 pound haddock
- 3 teaspoons water
- 2 tablespoons lemon juice
- Salt and black pepper to the taste
- 2 tablespoons mayonnaise
- 1 teaspoon dill, chopped
- Cooking spray
- ½ teaspoon old bay seasoning

Directions:
1. Spray your Slow cooker with the cooking spray, add lemon juice, water, fish, salt, pepper, mayo, dill and old bay seasoning, cover, cook on High for 2 hours.
2. Divide between plates and serve.

Nutrition: calories 274, fat 12, fiber 1, carbs 6, protein 20

Parsley Cod

Preparation time: 5 minutes
Cooking time: 2 hours
Servings: 2

Ingredients:
- 1 pound cod fillets, boneless
- 3 scallions, chopped
- 2 teaspoons olive oil
- Juice of 1 lime
- 1 teaspoon coriander, ground
- Salt and black pepper to the taste
- 1 tablespoon parsley, chopped

Directions:
1. In your slow cooker, mix the cod with the scallions, the oil and the other ingredients, rub gently, put the lid on and cook on High for 1 hour.
2. Divide everything between plates and serve.

Nutrition: calories 200, fat 12, fiber 2, carbs 6, protein 9

Buttery Trout

Preparation time: 10 minutes
Cooking time: 2 hours
Servings: 4

Ingredients:
- 4 trout fillets, boneless
- Salt and black pepper to the taste
- 3 teaspoons lemon zest, grated
- 3 tablespoons chives, chopped
- 6 tablespoons butter, melted
- 2 tablespoons olive oil
- 2 teaspoons lemon juice

Directions:
1. Put the butter in your Slow cooker, add trout fillets, season with salt, pepper, lemon zest, chives, oil and lemon juice, rub fish a bit, cover and cook on High for 2 hours.
2. Divide fish between plates and serve with the butter sauce drizzled on top.

Nutrition: calories 320, fat 12, fiber 6, carbs 12, protein 24

Pesto Cod and Tomatoes

Preparation time: 10 minutes
Cooking time: 3 hours
Servings: 2

Ingredients:
- 1 pound cod, boneless and roughly cubed
- 2 tablespoons basil pesto
- 1 tablespoon olive oil
- 1 cup cherry tomatoes, halved
- 1 tablespoon chives, chopped
- ½ cup veggie stock
- A pinch of salt and black pepper

Directions:
1. In your slow cooker, mix the cod with the pesto, oil and the other ingredients, toss, put the lid on and cook on High for 3 hours.
2. Divide the mix between plates and serve.

Nutrition: calories 211, fat 13, fiber 2, carbs 7, protein 11

Easy Salmon and Kimchi Sauce

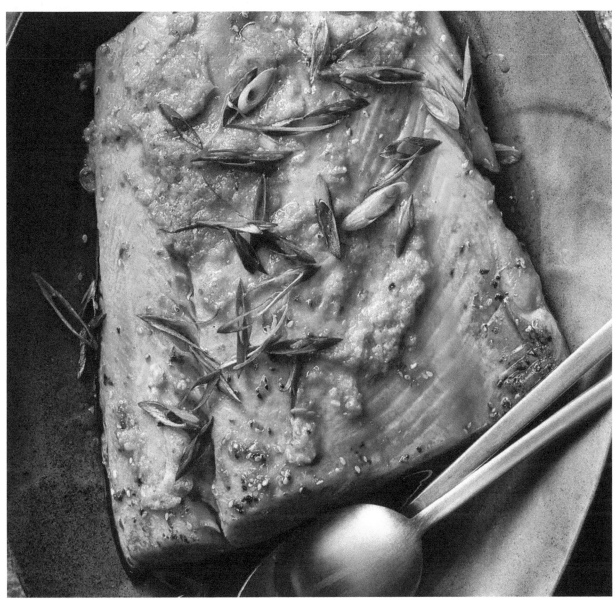

Preparation time: 10 minutes
Cooking time: 2 hours
Servings: 4

Ingredients:
- 2 tablespoons butter, soft
- 1 and ¼ pound salmon fillet
- 2 ounces Kimchi, finely chopped
- Salt and black pepper to the taste

Directions:

1. In your food processor, mix butter with Kimchi, blend well, rub salmon with salt, pepper and Kimchi mix, place in your Slow cooker, cover and cook on High for 2 hours.
2. Divide between plates and serve with a side salad.

Nutrition: calories 270, fat 12, fiber 5, carbs 13, protein 21

Orange Cod

Preparation time: 5 minutes
Cooking time: 3 hours
Servings: 2

Ingredients:
- 1 pound cod fillets, boneless
- Juice of 1 orange
- 1 tablespoon avocado oil
- 2 scallions, chopped
- ½ teaspoon turmeric powder
- ½ teaspoon sweet paprika
- A pinch of salt and black pepper

Directions:
1. In your slow cooker, mix the cod with the orange juice, oil and the other ingredients, toss, put the lid on and cook on High 3 hours.
2. Divide the mix between plates and serve.

Nutrition: calories 200, fat 12, fiber 4, carbs 6, protein 8

Salmon Meatballs and Sauce

Preparation time: 10 minutes
Cooking time: 2 hours
Servings: 4

Ingredients:
- 2 tablespoons butter
- 2 garlic cloves, minced
- 1/3 cup onion, chopped
- 1 pound wild salmon, boneless and minced
- ¼ cup chives, chopped
- 1 egg
- 2 tablespoons Dijon mustard
- 1 tablespoon flour
- Salt and black pepper to the taste

For the sauce:
- 4 garlic cloves, minced
- 2 tablespoons butter, melted
- 2 tablespoons Dijon mustard
- Juice and Zest of 1 lemon
- 2 cups coconut cream
- 2 tablespoons chives, chopped

Directions:
1. Heat up a pan with 2 tablespoons butter over medium heat, add onion and 2 garlic cloves, stir, cook for 3 minutes and transfer to a bowl.
2. In another bowl, mix onion and garlic with salmon, chives, flour, salt, pepper, 2 tablespoons mustard and egg and stir well.
3. Shape meatballs from the salmon mix and put them in your Slow cooker.
4. Add 2 tablespoons butter, 4 garlic cloves, coconut cream, 2 teaspoons mustard, lemon juice, lemon zest and chives, cover and cook on High for 2 hours.
5. Divide meatballs on plates, drizzle the sauce all over and serve.

Nutrition: calories 271, fat 5, fiber 1, carbs 6, protein 23

Garlic Sea Bass

Preparation time: 5 minutes
Cooking time: 4 hours
Servings: 2

Ingredients:
- 1 pound sea bass fillets, boneless
- 2 teaspoons avocado oil
- 3 garlic cloves, minced
- 1 green chili pepper, minced
- ½ teaspoon rosemary, dried
- ½ cup chicken stock
- A pinch of salt and black pepper
- 1 tablespoon cilantro, chopped

Directions:
1. In your slow cooker, mix the sea bass with the oil, garlic and the other ingredients, toss gently, put the lid on and cook on Low for 4 hours.
2. Divide the mix between plates and serve.

Nutrition: calories 232, fat 7, fiber 3, carbs 7, protein 9

Salmon and Caper Sauce

Preparation time: 10 minutes
Cooking time: 20 minutes
Servings: 3

Ingredients:
- 3 salmon fillets, boneless
- Salt and black pepper to the taste
- 1 tablespoon olive oil
- 1 tablespoon Italian seasoning
- 2 tablespoons capers
- 3 tablespoons lemon juice
- 4 garlic cloves, minced
- 2 tablespoons butter

Directions:
1. Put the butter in your Slow cooker, add salmon fillets, salt, pepper, oil, seasoning, capers, lemon juice and garlic, cover and cook on High for 2 hours.
2. Divide fish and sauce between plates and serve.

Nutrition: calories 245, fat 12, fiber 1, carbs 13, protein 23

Tuna and Brussels Sprouts

Preparation time: 5 minutes
Cooking time: 3 hours
Servings: 2

Ingredients:
- 1 pound tuna fillets, boneless
- ½ cup chicken stock
- 1 teaspoon sweet paprika
- ½ teaspoon chili powder
- 1 cup Brussels sprouts, trimmed and halved
- 1 red onion, chopped
- ½ teaspoon garlic powder
- A pinch of salt and black pepper
- 1 tablespoon cilantro, chopped

Directions:
1. In your slow cooker, mix the tuna with the stock, sprouts and the other ingredients, put the lid on and cook on High for 3 hours.
2. Divide the mix between plates and serve.

Nutrition: calories 232, fat 9, fiber 2, carbs 6, protein 8

Tabasco Halibut

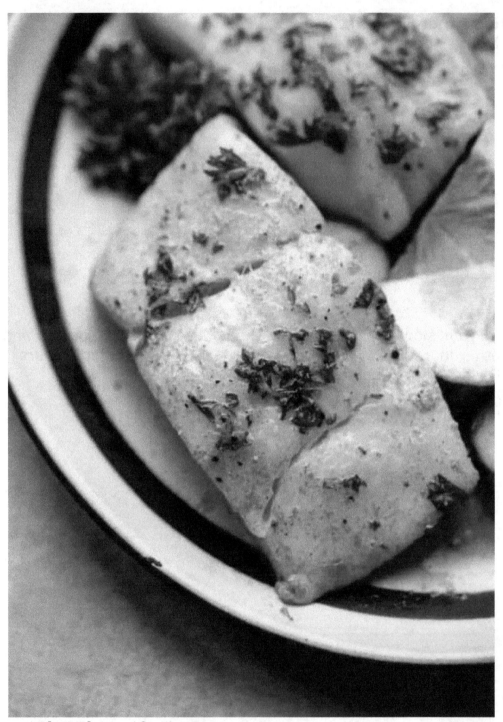

Preparation time: 10 minutes
Cooking time: 2 hours
Servings: 4

Ingredients:
- ½ cup parmesan, grated

- ¼ cup butter, melted
- ¼ cup mayonnaise
- 2 tablespoons green onions, chopped
- 6 garlic cloves, minced
- ½ teaspoon Tabasco sauce
- 4 halibut fillets, boneless
- Salt and black pepper to the taste
- Juice of ½ lemon

Directions:
1. Season halibut with salt, pepper and some of the lemon juice, place in your Slow cooker, add butter, mayo, green onions, garlic, Tabasco sauce and lemon juice, toss a bit, cover and cook on High for 2 hours.
2. Add parmesan, leave fish mix aside for a few more minutes, divide between plates and serve.

Nutrition: calories 240, fat 12, fiber 1, carbs 15, protein 23

Shrimp with Spinach

Preparation time: 10 minutes
Cooking time: 1 hour
Servings: 2

Ingredients:
- 1 pound shrimp, peeled and deveined
- 1 cup baby spinach
- ¼ cup tomato passata
- ½ cup chicken stock
- 3 scallions, chopped
- 1 tablespoon olive oil
- ½ teaspoon sweet paprika
- A pinch of salt and black pepper
- 1 tablespoon chives, chopped

Directions:
1. In your slow cooker, mix the shrimp with the spinach, tomato passata and the other ingredients, toss, put the lid on and cook on High for 1 hour.
2. Divide the mix between plates and serve.

Nutrition: calories 200, fat 13, fiber 3, carbs 6, protein 11

Creamy Salmon

Preparation time: 10 minutes
Cooking time: 2 hours
Servings: 4

Ingredients:
- 4 salmon fillets, boneless
- 1 tablespoon olive oil
- Salt and black pepper to the taste
- 1/3 cup parmesan, grated
- 1 and ½ teaspoon mustard
- ½ cup sour cream

Directions:
1. Place salmon in your Slow cooker, season with salt and pepper, drizzle the oil and rub.
2. In a bowl, mix sour cream with parmesan, mustard, salt and pepper, stir well, spoon this over the salmon fillets, cover and cook on High for 2 hours.
3. Divide between plates and serve.

Nutrition: calories 263, fat 6, fiber 1, carbs 14, protein 20

Shrimp and Avocado

Preparation time: 5 minutes
Cooking time: 1 hour
Servings: 2

Ingredients:
- 1 pound shrimp, peeled and deveined
- 1 cup avocado, peeled, pitted and cubed
- ½ cup chicken stock
- ½ teaspoon sweet paprika
- Juice of 1 lime
- 1 tablespoon olive oil
- 2 tablespoons chili pepper, minced
- A pinch of salt and black pepper
- 1 tablespoon chives, chopped

Directions:
1. In your slow cooker, mix the shrimp with the avocado, stock and the other ingredients, toss, put the lid on and cook on High for 1 hour.
2. Divide the mix into bowls and serve.

Nutrition: calories 490, fat 25.4, fiber 5.8, carbs 11.9, protein 53.6

Chinese Cod

Preparation time: 10 minutes
Cooking time: 2 hours
Servings: 4

Ingredients:
- 1 pound cod, cut into medium pieces
- Salt and black pepper to the taste
- 2 green onions, chopped
- 3 garlic cloves, minced
- 3 tablespoons soy sauce
- 1 cup fish stock
- 1 tablespoons balsamic vinegar
- 1 tablespoon ginger, grated
- ½ teaspoon chili pepper, crushed

Directions:
1. In your Slow cooker, mix fish with salt, pepper green onions, garlic, soy sauce, fish stock, vinegar, ginger and chili pepper, toss, cover and cook on High for 2 hours.
2. Divide everything between plates and serve.

Nutrition: calories 204, fat 3, fiber 6, carbs 14, protein 24

Chives Mackerel

Preparation time: 10 minutes
Cooking time: 4 hours
Servings: 2

Ingredients:
- 1 pound mackerel fillets, boneless
- ½ teaspoon cumin, ground
- ½ teaspoon coriander, ground
- 2 garlic cloves, minced
- 1 tablespoon avocado oil
- 1 tablespoon lime juice
- ½ cup chicken stock
- A pinch of salt and black pepper
- 2 tablespoons chives, chopped

Directions:
1. In your slow cooker, mix the mackerel with the cumin, coriander and the other ingredients, put the lid on and cook on Low for 4 hours.
2. Divide the mix between plates and serve with a side salad.

Nutrition: calories 613, fat 41.6, fiber 0.5, carbs 2, protein 54.7

Fish Mix

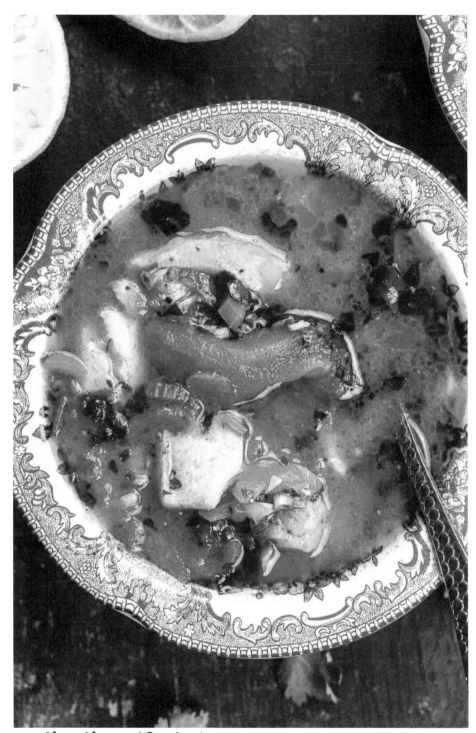

Preparation time: 10 minutes
Cooking time: 2 hours and 30 minutes
Servings: 4

Ingredients:

- 4 white fish fillets, skinless and boneless
- ½ teaspoon mustard seeds
- Salt and black pepper to the taste
- 2 green chilies, chopped
- 1 teaspoon ginger, grated
- 1 teaspoon curry powder
- ¼ teaspoon cumin, ground
- 2 tablespoons olive oil
- 1 small red onion, chopped
- 1-inch turmeric root, grated
- ¼ cup cilantro, chopped
- 1 and ½ cups coconut cream
- 3 garlic cloves, minced

Directions:
1. Heat up a slow cooker with half of the oil over medium heat, add mustard seeds, ginger, onion, garlic, turmeric, chilies, curry powder and cumin, stir and cook for 3-4 minutes.
2. Add the rest of the oil to your Slow cooker, add spice mix, fish, coconut milk, salt and pepper, cover and cook on High for 2 hours and 30 minutes.
3. Divide into bowls and serve with the cilantro sprinkled on top.

Nutrition: calories 500, fat 34, fiber 7, carbs 13, protein 44

Dill Cod

Preparation time: 10 minutes
Cooking time: 3 hours
Servings: 2

Ingredients:
- 1 tablespoon olive oil
- 1 pound cod fillets, boneless and cubed
- 1 tablespoon dill, chopped
- ½ teaspoon sweet paprika
- ½ teaspoon cumin, ground
- 2 garlic cloves, minced
- 1 teaspoon lemon juice
- 1 cup tomato passata
- A pinch of salt and black pepper

Directions:
1. In your slow cooker, mix the cod with the oil, dill and the other ingredients, toss, put the lid on and cook on Low for 3 hours.
2. Divide the mix between plates and serve.

Nutrition: calories 192, fat 9, fiber 2, carbs 8, protein 7

Italian Barramundi and Tomato Relish

Preparation time: 10 minutes
Cooking time: 2 hours
Servings: 4

Ingredients:
- 2 barramundi fillets, skinless
- 2 teaspoon olive oil
- 2 teaspoons Italian seasoning
- ¼ cup green olives, pitted and chopped
- ¼ cup cherry tomatoes, chopped
- ¼ cup black olives, chopped
- 1 tablespoon lemon zest
- 2 tablespoons lemon zest
- Salt and black pepper to the taste
- 2 tablespoons parsley, chopped
- 1 tablespoon olive oil

Directions:
1. Rub fish with salt, pepper, Italian seasoning and 2 teaspoons olive oil and put into your Slow cooker.
2. In a bowl, mix tomatoes with all the olives, salt, pepper, lemon zest and lemon juice, parsley and 1 tablespoon olive oil, toss, add over fish, cover and cook on High for 2 hours.
3. Divide fish between plates, top with tomato relish and serve.

Nutrition: calories 140, fat 4, fiber 2, carbs 11, protein 10

Shrimp and Mango Mix

Preparation time: 10 minutes
Cooking time: 1 hour
Servings: 2

Ingredients:
- 1 pound shrimp, peeled and deveined
- ½ cup mango, peeled and cubed
- ½ cup cherry tomatoes, halved
- ½ cup shallots, chopped
- 1 tablespoon lime juice
- ½ teaspoon rosemary, dried
- 1 tablespoon olive oil
- ½ teaspoon chili powder
- ½ cup chicken stock
- A pinch of salt and black pepper
- 1 tablespoon chives, chopped

Directions:
1. In your slow cooker, mix the shrimp with the mango, tomatoes and the other ingredients, toss, put the lid on and cook on High for 1 hour.
2. Divide the mix into bowls and serve.

Nutrition: calories 210, fat 9, fiber 2, carbs 6, protein 7

Spicy Creole Shrimp

Preparation time: 10 minutes
Cooking time: 1 hour and 30 minutes
Servings: 2

Ingredients:
- ½ pound big shrimp, peeled and deveined
- 2 teaspoons Worcestershire sauce
- 2 teaspoons olive oil
- Juice of 1 lemon
- Salt and black pepper to the taste
- 1 teaspoon Creole seasoning

Directions:
1. In your Slow cooker, mix shrimp with Worcestershire sauce, oil, lemon juice, salt, pepper and Creole seasoning, toss, cover and cook on High for 1 hour and 30 minutes.
2. Divide into bowls and serve.

Nutrition: calories 140, fat 3, fiber 1, carbs 6, protein 6

Balsamic Tuna

Preparation time: 5 minutes
Cooking time: 3 hours
Servings: 2

Ingredients:
- 1 pound tuna fillets, boneless and roughly cubed
- 1 tablespoon balsamic vinegar
- 3 garlic cloves, minced
- 1 tablespoon avocado oil
- ¼ cup chicken stock
- 1 tablespoon hives, chopped
- A pinch of salt and black pepper

Directions:
1. In your slow cooker, mix the tuna with the garlic, vinegar and the other ingredients, toss, put the lid on and cook on Low for 3 hours.
2. Divide the mix into bowls and serve.

Nutrition: calories 200, fat 10, fiber 2, carbs 5, protein 9

Sriracha Shrimp

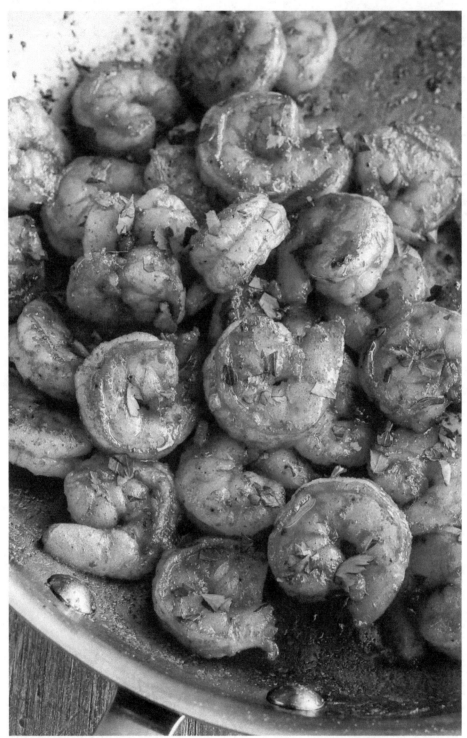

Preparation time: 10 minutes
Cooking time: 1 hour and 30 minutes
Servings: 6

Ingredients:

- ¼ cup yellow onion, chopped
- 2 tablespoons olive oil
- 1 garlic clove, minced
- 1 and ½ pounds shrimp, peeled and deveined
- ¼ cup red pepper, roasted and chopped
- 14 ounces canned tomatoes, chopped
- ¼ cup cilantro, chopped
- 2 tablespoons sriracha sauce
- 1 cup coconut milk
- Salt and black pepper to the taste
- 2 tablespoons lime juice

Directions:
1. Put the oil in your Slow cooker, add onion, garlic, shrimp, red pepper, tomatoes, cilantro, sriracha sauce, milk, salt, pepper and lime juice, toss, cover and cook on High for 1 hour and 30 minutes.
2. Divide into bowls and serve.

Nutrition: calories 250, fat 12, fiber 3, carbs 5, protein 20

Lime Trout Mix

Preparation time: 10 minutes
Cooking time: 2 hours
Servings: 2

Ingredients:
- 1 pound trout fillets, boneless
- 1 tablespoon olive oil
- ½ cup chicken stock
- 2 tablespoons lime zest, grated
- 2 tablespoons lemon juice
- 1 teaspoon garam masala
- A pinch of salt and black pepper

Directions:
1. In your slow cooker, mix the trout with the olive oil, lime juice and the other ingredients, toss, put the lid on and cook on High for 2 hours.
2. Divide everything between plates and serve.

Nutrition: calories 200, fat 13, fiber 3, carbs 6, protein 11

Shrimp and Peas Soup

Preparation time: 10 minutes
Cooking time: 1 hour
Servings: 4

Ingredients:
- 4 scallions, chopped
- 1 tablespoon olive oil
- 1 small ginger root, grated
- 8 cups chicken stock
- ¼ cup soy sauce
- 5 ounces canned bamboo shoots, sliced
- Black pepper to the taste
- ¼ teaspoon fish sauce
- 1 pound shrimp, peeled and deveined
- ½ pound snow peas
- 1 tablespoon sesame oil
- ½ tablespoon chili oil

Directions:
1. In your Slow cooker, mix olive oil with scallions, ginger, stock, soy sauce, bamboo, black pepper, fish sauce, shrimp, peas, sesame oil and chili oil, cover and cook on High for 1 hour.
2. Stir soup, ladle into bowls and serve.

Nutrition: calories 240, fat 3, fiber 2, carbs 12, protein 14

Creamy Tuna and Scallions

Preparation time: 10 minutes
Cooking time: 2 hours
Servings: 2

Ingredients:
- 1 pound tuna fillets, boneless and cubed
- 4 scallions, chopped
- ½ cup heavy cream
- ½ cup chicken stock
- 1 tablespoon olive oil
- 1 teaspoon turmeric powder
- A pinch of salt and black pepper
- 1 tablespoon chives, chopped

Directions:
1. In your slow cooker, mix the tuna with the scallions, cream and the other ingredients, toss, put the lid on and cook on High for 2 hours.
2. Divide the mix into bowls and serve.

Nutrition: calories 198, fat 7, fiber 2, carbs 6, protein 7

Calamari and Sauce

Preparation time: 10 minutes
Cooking time: 2 hours and 20 minutes
Servings: 2

Ingredients:
- 1 squid, cut into medium rings
- A pinch of cayenne pepper
- 2 tablespoons flour
- Salt and black pepper to the taste
- ¼ cup fish stock
- 1 tablespoons lemon juice
- 4 tablespoons mayo
- 1 teaspoon sriracha sauce

Directions:
1. Season squid rings with salt, pepper and cayenne and put them in your Slow cooker.
2. Add flour, stock, lemon juice and sriracha sauce, toss, cover and cook on High for 2 hour and 20 minutes.
3. Add mayo, toss, divide between plates and serve.

Nutrition: calories 345, fat 32, fiber 3, carbs 12, protein 13

Cod and Mustard Sauce

Preparation time: 10 minutes
Cooking time: 3 hours
Servings: 2

Ingredients:
- 1 tablespoon olive oil
- 1 pound cod fillets, boneless
- 2 tablespoons mustard
- ½ cup heavy cream
- ¼ cup chicken stock
- 2 garlic cloves, minced
- A pinch of salt and black pepper
- 1 tablespoon chives, chopped

Directions:
1. In your slow cooker, mix the cod with the oil, mustard and the other ingredients, toss gently, put the lid on and cook on Low for 3 hours.
2. Divide the mix between plates and serve.

Nutrition: calories 221, fat 8, fiber 3, carbs 6, protein 7

Calamari and Shrimp

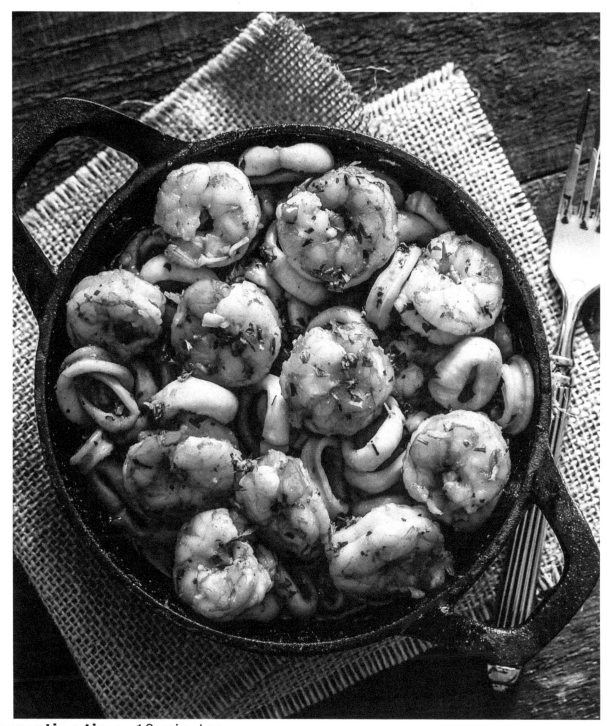

Preparation time: 10 minutes
Cooking time: 2 hours and 30 minutes
Servings: 2

Ingredients:

- 8 ounces calamari, cut into medium rings
- 7 ounces shrimp, peeled and deveined
- 3 tablespoons flour
- 1 tablespoon olive oil
- 2 tablespoons avocado, chopped
- 1 teaspoon tomato paste
- 1 tablespoon mayonnaise
- 1 teaspoon Worcestershire sauce
- 1 teaspoon lemon juice
- 2 lemon slices
- Salt and black pepper to the taste
- ½ teaspoon turmeric powder

Directions:
1. In your Slow cooker, mix calamari with flour, oil, tomato paste, mayo, Worcestershire sauce, lemon juice, lemon slices, salt, pepper and turmeric, cover and cook on High for 2 hours.
2. Add shrimp, cover and cook on High for 30 minutes more.
3. Divide between plates and serve.

Nutrition: calories 368, fat 23, fiber 3, carbs 10, protein 34

Shrimp and Pineapple Bowls

Preparation time: 5 minutes
Cooking time: 1 hour
Servings: 2

Ingredients:
- 1 pound shrimp, peeled and deveined
- 1 cup pineapple, peeled and cubed
- 1 teaspoon sweet paprika
- 1 tablespoon avocado oil
- 3 scallions, chopped
- ½ cup chicken stock
- A pinch of salt and black pepper

Directions:
1. In your slow cooker, mix the shrimp with the pineapple, paprika and the other ingredients, toss, put the lid on and cook on High for 1 hour.
2. Divide the mix into bowls and serve.

Nutrition: calories 235, fat 8, fiber 4, carbs 7, protein 9

Clam Chowder

Preparation time: 10 minutes
Cooking time: 2 hours
Servings: 4

Ingredients:
- 1 cup celery stalks, chopped
- Salt and black pepper to the taste
- 1 teaspoon thyme, ground
- 2 cups chicken stock
- 14 ounces canned baby clams
- 2 cups whipping cream
- 1 cup onion, chopped
- 13 bacon slices, chopped

Directions:
1. Heat up a pan over medium heat, add bacon slices, brown them and transfer to a bowl.
2. Heat up the same pan over medium heat, add celery and onion, stir and cook for 5 minutes.
3. Transfer everything to your Slow cooker, also add bacon, baby clams, salt, pepper, stock, thyme and whipping cream, stir and cook on High for 2 hours.
4. Divide into bowls and serve.

Nutrition: calories 420, fat 22, fiber 0, carbs 5, protein 25

Lime Crab

Preparation time: 10 minutes
Cooking time: 2 hours
Servings: 2

Ingredients:
- 1 tablespoon avocado oil
- 1 pound crab meat
- ¼ cup shallots, chopped
- 1 tablespoon lime juice
- ½ cup fish stock
- 1 teaspoon sweet paprika
- 1 tablespoon chives, chopped
- A pinch of salt and black pepper

Directions:
1. In your slow cooker, mix the crab with the oil, shallots and the other ingredients, toss, put the lid on and cook on High for 2 hours.
2. Divide everything into bowls and serve.

Nutrition: calories 211, fat 8, fiber 4, carbs 8, protein 8

Shrimp Salad
Preparation time: 10 minutes
Cooking time: 1 hour
Servings: 4

Ingredients:
- 2 tablespoons olive oil
- 1 pound shrimp, peeled and deveined
- Salt and black pepper to the taste
- 2 tablespoons lime juice
- 3 endives, leaves separated
- 3 tablespoons parsley, chopped
- 2 teaspoons mint, chopped
- 1 tablespoon tarragon, chopped
- 1 tablespoon lemon juice
- 2 tablespoons mayonnaise
- 1 teaspoon lime zest
- ½ cup sour cream

Directions:
1. In a bowl, mix shrimp with salt, pepper and the olive oil, toss to coat and spread into the Slow cooker,
2. Add lime juice, endives, parsley, mint, tarragon, lemon juice, lemon zest, mayo and sour cream, toss, cover and cook on High for 1 hour.
3. Divide into bowls and serve.

Nutrition: calories 200, fat 11, fiber 2, carbs 11, protein 13

Hot Salmon and Carrots

Preparation time: 10 minutes
Cooking time: 3 hours
Servings: 2

Ingredients:
- 1 pound salmon fillets, boneless
- 1 cup baby carrots, peeled
- ½ teaspoon hot paprika
- ½ teaspoon chili powder
- ¼ cup chicken stock
- 2 scallions, chopped
- 1 tablespoon smoked paprika
- A pinch of salt and black pepper
- 2 tablespoons chives, chopped

Directions:
1. In your slow cooker, mix the salmon with the carrots, paprika and the other ingredients, toss, put the lid on and cook on Low for 3 hours.
2. Divide the mix between plates and serve.

Nutrition: calories 193, fat 7, fiber 3, carbs 6, protein 6

Italian Clams

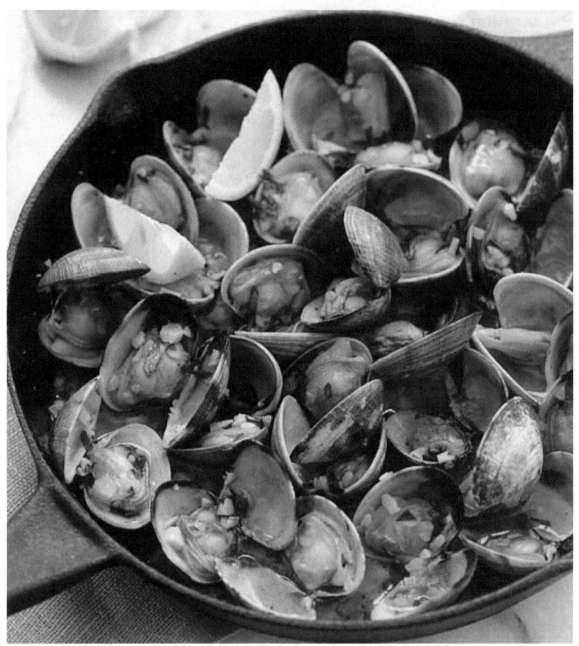

Preparation time: 10 minutes
Cooking time: 2 hours
Servings: 6

Ingredients:
- ½ cup butter, melted
- 36 clams, scrubbed
- 1 teaspoon red pepper flakes, crushed
- 1 teaspoon parsley, chopped

- 5 garlic cloves, minced
- 1 tablespoon oregano, dried
- 2 cups white wine

Directions:
1. In your Slow cooker, mix butter with clams, pepper flakes, parsley, garlic, oregano and wine, stir, cover and cook on High for 2 hours.
2. Divide into bowls and serve.

Nutrition: calories 224, fat 15, fiber 2, carbs 7, protein 4

Shrimp and Eggplant

Preparation time: 5 minutes
Cooking time: 1 hour
Servings: 2

Ingredients:
- 1 pound shrimp, peeled and deveined
- 2 teaspoons avocado oil
- 1 eggplant, cubed
- 2 tomatoes, cubed
- Juice of 1 lime
- ½ cup chicken stock
- 4 garlic cloves, minced
- 1 tablespoon coriander, chopped
- 1 tablespoon chives, chopped
- A pinch of salt and black pepper

Directions:
1. In your slow cooker, mix the shrimp with the oil, eggplant, tomatoes and the other ingredients, toss, put the lid on and cook on High for 1 hour.
2. Divide the mix into bowls and serve.

Nutrition: calories 200, fat 11, fiber 4, carbs 5, protein 12

Orange Salmon

Preparation time: 10 minutes
Cooking time: 2 hours
Servings: 2

Ingredients:
- 2 lemons, sliced
- 1 pound wild salmon, skinless and cubed
- ¼ cup balsamic vinegar
- ¼ cup red orange juice
- 1 teaspoon olive oil
- 1/3 cup orange marmalade

Directions:
1. Heat up a slow cooker over medium heat, add vinegar, orange juice and marmalade, stir well, bring to a simmer for 1 minute and transfer to your Slow cooker.
2. Add salmon, lemon slices and oil, toss, cover and cook on High for 2 hours.
3. Divide salmon plates and serve with a side salad.

Nutrition: calories 260, fat 3, fiber 2, carbs 16, protein 8

Sea Bass and Squash

Preparation time: 10 minutes
Cooking time: 3 hours
Servings: 2

Ingredients:
- 1 pound sea bass, boneless and cubed
- 1 cup butternut squash, peeled and cubed
- 1 teaspoon olive oil
- ½ teaspoon turmeric powder
- ½ teaspoon Italian seasoning
- 1 cup chicken stock
- 1 tablespoon cilantro, chopped

Directions:
1. In your slow cooker, mix the sea bass with the squash, oil, turmeric and the other ingredients, toss, the lid on and cook on Low for 3 hours.
2. Divide everything between plates and serve.

Nutrition: calories 200, fat 12, fiber 3, carbs 7, protein 9

Tuna and Chimichurri

Preparation time: 10 minutes
Cooking time: 1 hour and 15 minutes
Servings: 4

Ingredients:
- ½ cup cilantro, chopped
- 1/3 cup olive oil
- 1 small red onion, chopped
- 3 tablespoon balsamic vinegar
- 2 tablespoons parsley, chopped
- 2 tablespoons basil, chopped
- 1 jalapeno pepper, chopped
- 1 pound tuna steak, boneless, skinless and cubed
- Salt and black pepper to the taste
- 1 teaspoon red pepper flakes
- 2 garlic cloves, minced
- 1 teaspoon thyme, chopped
- A pinch of cayenne pepper
- 2 avocados, pitted, peeled and sliced
- 6 ounces baby arugula

Directions:
1. In a bowl, mix the oil with jalapeno, vinegar, onion, cilantro, basil, garlic, parsley, pepper flakes, thyme, cayenne, salt and pepper, whisk well, transfer to your Slow cooker, cover and cook on High for 1 hour.
2. Add tuna, cover and cook on High for 15 minutes more.
3. Divide arugula on plates, top with tuna slices, drizzle the chimichurri sauce and serve with avocado slices on the side.

Nutrition: calories 186, fat 3, fiber 1, carbs 4, protein 20

Coconut Mackerel

Preparation time: 5 minutes
Cooking time: 3 hours
Servings: 2

Ingredients:
- 1 pound mackerel fillets, boneless, skinless and cubed
- 1 tablespoon avocado oil
- 1 cup coconut cream
- ½ teaspoon cumin, ground
- 2 scallions, chopped
- A pinch of salt and black pepper
- ½ teaspoon garam masala
- 1 tablespoon cilantro, chopped

Directions:
1. In your slow cooker, mix the mackerel with the oil, cream and the other ingredients, toss, put the lid on and cook on Low for 3 hours.
2. Divide the mix into bowls and serve.

Nutrition: calories 232, fat 10, fiber 4, carbs 6, protein 9

Cider Clams

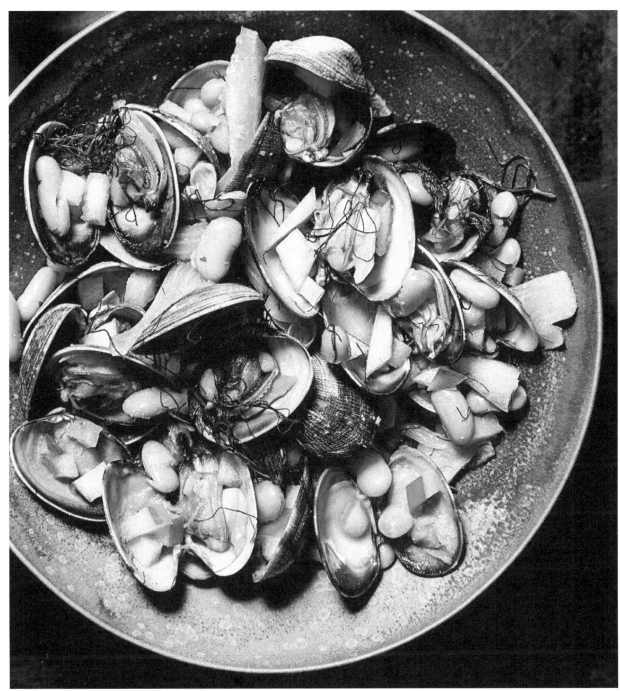

Preparation time: 10 minutes
Cooking time: 2 hours
Servings: 4

Ingredients:
- 2 pounds clams, scrubbed
- 3 ounces pancetta

- 1 tablespoon olive oil
- 3 tablespoons butter, melted
- 2 garlic cloves, minced
- 1 bottle infused cider
- Salt and black pepper to the taste
- Juice of ½ lemon
- 1 small green apple, chopped
- 2 thyme springs, chopped

Directions:
1. Heat up a pan with the oil over medium-high heat, add pancetta, brown for 3 minutes and transfer to your Slow cooker.
2. Add butter, garlic, salt, pepper, shallot, cider, clams, thyme, lemon juice and apple, cover and cook on High for 2 hours.
3. Divide everything into bowls and serve.

Nutrition: calories 270, fat 2, fiber 1, carbs 11, protein 20

Salmon and Peas

Preparation time: 10 minutes
Cooking time: 2 hours
Servings: 2

Ingredients:
- 1 pound salmon fillets, boneless and cubed
- 1 tablespoon olive oil
- 1 cup sugar snap peas
- 1 tablespoon lemon juice
- ½ cup tomato passata
- 1 tablespoon chives, chopped
- Salt and black pepper to the taste

Directions:
1. In your slow cooker, mix the salmon with the peas, oil and the other ingredients, toss, put the lid on and cook on High for 2 hour.
2. Divide the mix between plates and serve.

Nutrition: calories 182, fat 7, fiber 3, carbs 6, protein 9

Mustard Salmon

Preparation time: 10 minutes
Cooking time: 2 hours
Servings: 1

Ingredients:
- 1 big salmon fillet
- Salt and black pepper to the taste
- 2 tablespoons mustard
- 1 tablespoon olive oil
- 1 tablespoon maple extract

Directions:
1. In a bowl, mix maple extract with mustard and whisk well.
2. Season salmon with salt and pepper, brush with the mustard mix, put in your Slow cooker, cover and cook on High for 2 hours.
3. Serve the salmon with a side salad.

Nutrition: calories 240, fat 7, fiber 1, carbs 15, protein 23

Chili Shrimp and Zucchinis

Preparation time: 10 minutes
Cooking time: 1 hour
Servings: 4

Ingredients:
- 1 pound shrimp, peeled and deveined
- 1 zucchini, cubed
- 2 scallions, minced
- 1 cup tomato passata
- 2 green chilies, chopped
- A pinch of salt and black pepper
- 1 tablespoon chives, chopped

Directions:
1. In your slow cooker, mix the shrimp with the zucchini and the other ingredients, toss, put the lid on and cook on High for 1 hour.
2. Divide the shrimp mix into bowls and serve.

Nutrition: calories 210, fat 8, fiber 3, carbs 6, protein 14

Salmon and Relish

Preparation time: 10 minutes
Cooking time: 2 hours
Servings: 2

Ingredients:
- 2 medium salmon fillets, boneless
- Salt and black pepper to the taste
- 1 shallot, chopped
- 1 tablespoon lemon juice
- 1 big lemon, peeled and cut into wedges
- ¼ cup olive oil+ 1 teaspoon
- 2 tablespoons parsley, finely chopped

Directions:
1. Brush salmon fillets with the olive oil, sprinkle with salt and pepper, put in your Slow cooker, add shallot and lemon juice, cover and cook on High for 2 hours.
2. Shed salmon and divide into 2 bowls.
3. Add lemon segments to your Slow cooker, also add ¼ cup oil and parsley and whisk well.
4. Divide this mix over salmon, toss and serve.

Nutrition: calories 200, fat 10, fiber 1, carbs 5, protein 20

Italian Shrimp

Preparation time: 5 minutes
Cooking time: 1 hour
Servings: 2

Ingredients:
- 1 pound shrimp, peeled and deveined
- 1 tablespoon avocado oil
- ½ teaspoon sweet paprika
- 1 teaspoon Italian seasoning
- Salt and black pepper to the taste
- Juice of 1 lime
- ¼ cup chicken stock
- 1 tablespoon chives, chopped

Directions:
1. In your slow cooker, mix the shrimp with the oil, seasoning and the other ingredients, toss, put the lid on and cook on High for 1 hour.
2. Divide the mix into bowls and serve.

Nutrition: calories 200, fat 12, fiber 3, carbs 6, protein 11

Mussels Soup

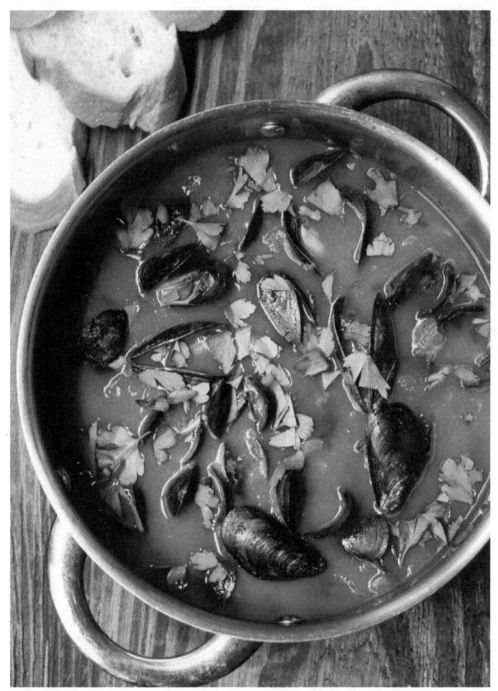

Preparation time: 10 minutes
Cooking time: 2 hours
Servings: 6

Ingredients:
- 2 pounds mussels
- 28 ounces canned tomatoes, crushed

- 28 ounces canned tomatoes, chopped
- 2 cup chicken stock
- 1 teaspoon red pepper flakes, crushed
- 3 garlic cloves, minced
- 1 handful parsley, chopped
- 1 yellow onion, chopped
- Salt and black pepper to the taste
- 1 tablespoon olive oil

Directions:

1. In your Slow cooker, mix mussels with canned and crushed tomatoes, stock, pepper flakes, garlic, parsley, onion, salt, pepper and oil, stir, cover and cook on High for 2 hours.
2. Divide into bowls and serve.

Nutrition: calories 250, fat 3, fiber 3, carbs 8, protein 12

Basil Cod and Olives

Preparation time: 5 minutes
Cooking time: 3 hours
Servings: 2

Ingredients:
- 1 pound cod fillets, boneless
- 1 cup black olives, pitted and halved
- ½ tablespoon tomato paste
- 1 tablespoon basil, chopped
- ¼ cup chicken stock
- 1 red onion, sliced
- 1 tablespoon lime juice
- 1 tablespoon chives, chopped
- Salt and black pepper to the taste

Directions:
1. In your slow cooker, mix the cod with the olives, basil and the other ingredients, toss, put the lid on and cook on Low for 3 hours.
2. Divide everything between plates and serve.

Nutrition: calories 132, fat 9, fiber 2, carbs 5, protein 11 Fish and Olives Mix

Indian Fish

Preparation time: 10 minutes
Cooking time: 2 hours
Servings: 6

Ingredients:
- 6 white fish fillets, cut into medium pieces
- 1 tomato, chopped
- 14 ounces coconut milk
- 2 yellow onions, sliced
- 2 red bell peppers, cut into strips
- 2 garlic cloves, minced
- 6 curry leaves
- 1 tablespoons coriander, ground
- 1 tablespoon ginger, finely grated
- ½ teaspoon turmeric, ground
- 2 teaspoons cumin, ground
- Salt and black pepper to the taste
- ½ teaspoon fenugreek, ground
- 1 teaspoon hot pepper flakes
- 2 tablespoons lemon juice

Directions:
1. In your Slow cooker, mix fish with tomato, milk, onions, bell peppers, garlic cloves, curry leaves, coriander, turmeric, cumin, salt, pepper, fenugreek, pepper flakes and lemon juice, cover and cook on High for 2 hours.
2. Toss fish, divide the whole mix between plates and serve.

Nutrition: calories 231, fat 4, fiber 6, carbs 16, protein 22

Tuna and Fennel

Preparation time: 10 minutes
Cooking time: 2 hours
Servings: 2

Ingredients:
- 1 pound tuna fillets, boneless and cubed
- 1 fennel bulb, sliced
- ½ cup chicken stock
- ½ teaspoon sweet paprika
- ½ teaspoon chili powder
- 1 red onion, chopped
- A pinch of salt and black pepper
- 2 tablespoons cilantro, chopped

Directions:
1. In your slow cooker, mix the tuna with the fennel, stock and the other ingredients, toss, put the lid on and cook on High for 2 hour.
2. Divide the mix between plates and serve.

Nutrition: calories 200, fat 12, fiber 2, carbs 6, protein 11

Cod and Peas

Preparation time: 15 minutes
Cooking time: 2 hours
Servings: 4

Ingredients:
- 16 ounces cod fillets
- 1 tablespoon parsley, chopped
- 10 ounces peas
- 9 ounces wine
- ½ teaspoon oregano, dried
- ½ teaspoon paprika
- 2 garlic cloves, chopped
- Salt and pepper to the taste

Directions:
1. In your food processor mix garlic with parsley, oregano, paprika and wine, blend well and add to your Slow cooker.
2. Add fish, peas, salt and pepper, cover and cook on High for 2 hours.
3. Divide into bowls and serve.

Nutrition: calories 251, far 2, fiber 6, carbs 7, protein 22

Shrimp and Mushrooms

Preparation time: 10 minutes
Cooking time: 1 hour
Servings: 2

Ingredients:
- 1 pound shrimp, peeled and deveined
- 1 cup white mushrooms, halved
- 1 tablespoon avocado oil
- ½ tablespoon tomato paste
- 4 scallions, minced
- ½ cup chicken stock
- Juice of 1 lime
- Salt and black pepper to the taste
- 1 tablespoon chives, minced

Directions:
1. In your slow cooker, mix the shrimp with the mushrooms, oil and the other ingredients, toss, put the lid on and cook on High for 1 hour.
2. Divide the mix into bowls and serve.

Nutrition: calories 200, fat 12, fiber 2, carbs 6, protein 9

Salmon and Rice

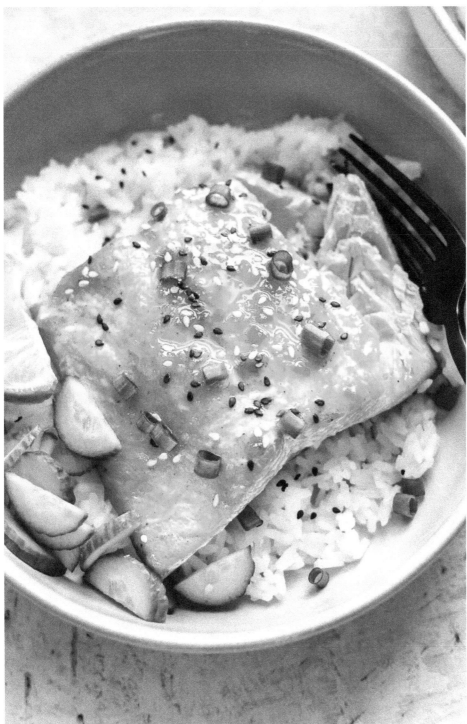

Preparation time: 5 minutes
Cooking time: 2 hours
Servings: 2

Ingredients:

- 2 wild salmon fillets, boneless
- Salt and black pepper to the taste
- ½ cup jasmine rice
- 1 cup chicken stock
- ¼ cup veggie stock
- 1 tablespoon butter
- A pinch of saffron

Directions:
1. In your Slow cooker mix stock with rice, stock, butter and saffron and stir.
2. Add salmon, salt and pepper, cover and cook on High for 2 hours.
3. Divide salmon on plates, add rice mix on the side and serve.

Nutrition: calories 312, fat 4, fiber 6, carbs 20, protein 22

Salmon and Berries

Preparation time: 10 minutes
Cooking time: 3 hours
Servings: 2

Ingredients:
- 1 pound salmon fillets, boneless and roughly cubed
- ½ cup blackberries
- Juice of 1 lime
- 1 tablespoon avocado oil
- 2 scallions, chopped
- ½ teaspoon Italian seasoning
- ½ cup fish stock
- A pinch of salt and black pepper

Directions:
1. In your slow cooker, mix the salmon with the berries, lime juice and the other ingredients, toss, put the lid on and cook on Low for 3 hours.
2. Divide the mix between plates and serve.

Nutrition: calories 211, fat 13, fiber 2, carbs 7, protein 11

Milky Fish

Preparation time: 10 minutes
Cooking time: 2 hours
Servings: 6

Ingredients:
- 17 ounces white fish, skinless, boneless and cut into medium chunks
- 1 yellow onion, chopped
- 13 ounces potatoes, peeled and cut into chunks
- 13 ounces milk
- Salt and black pepper to the taste
- 14 ounces chicken stock
- 14 ounces water
- 14 ounces half and half

Directions:
1. In your Slow cooker, mix fish with onion, potatoes, water, milk and stock, cover and cook on High for 2 hours.
2. Add salt, pepper, half and half, stir, divide into bowls and serve.

Nutrition: calories 203, fat 4, fiber 5, carbs 20, protein 15

Cod and Artichokes

Preparation time: 5 minutes
Cooking time: 3 hours
Servings: 2

Ingredients:
- 1 pound cod fillets, boneless and roughly cubed
- 1 cup canned artichoke hearts, drained and quartered
- 2 scallions, chopped
- 1 tablespoon olive oil
- ½ cup chicken stock
- 1 tablespoon lime juice
- 1 tablespoon cilantro, chopped
- A pinch of salt and black pepper

Directions:
1. In your slow cooker, mix the cod with the artichokes, scallions and the other ingredients, toss, put the lid on and cook on Low for 3 hours.
2. Divide the mix between plates and serve.

Nutrition: calories 200, fat 12, fiber 4, carbs 6, protein 8

Salmon and Raspberry Vinaigrette

Preparation time: 2 hours
Cooking time: 2 hours
Servings: 6

Ingredients:
- 6 salmon steaks
- 2 tablespoons olive oil
- 4 leeks, sliced
- 2 garlic cloves, minced
- 2 tablespoons parsley, chopped
- 1 cup clam juice
- 2 tablespoons lemon juice
- Salt and white pepper to the taste
- 1 teaspoon sherry
- 1/3 cup dill, chopped

For the raspberry vinegar:
- 2 pints red raspberries
- 1-pint cider vinegar

Directions:
1. In a bowl, mix red raspberries with vinegar and salmon, toss, cover and keep in the fridge for 2 hours.
2. In your Slow cooker, mix oil with parsley, leeks, garlic, clam juice, lemon juice, salt, pepper, sherry, dill and salmon, cover and cook on High for 2 hours.
3. Divide everything between plates and serve.

Nutrition: calories 251, fat 6, fiber 7, carbs 16, protein 26

Salmon, Tomatoes and Green Beans

Preparation time: 5 minutes
Cooking time: 2 hours
Servings: 2

Ingredients:
- 1 pound salmon fillets, boneless and cubed
- 1 cup cherry tomatoes, halved
- 1 cup green beans, trimmed and halved
- 1 cup tomato passata
- ½ cup chicken stock
- A pinch of salt and black pepper
- 1 tablespoon parsley, chopped

Directions:
1. In your slow cooker, mix the salmon with the tomatoes, green beans and the other ingredients, toss, put the lid on and cook on High for 2 hours.
2. Divide the mix into bowls and serve.

Nutrition: calories 232, fat 7, fiber 3, carbs 7, protein 9

Fish Pudding

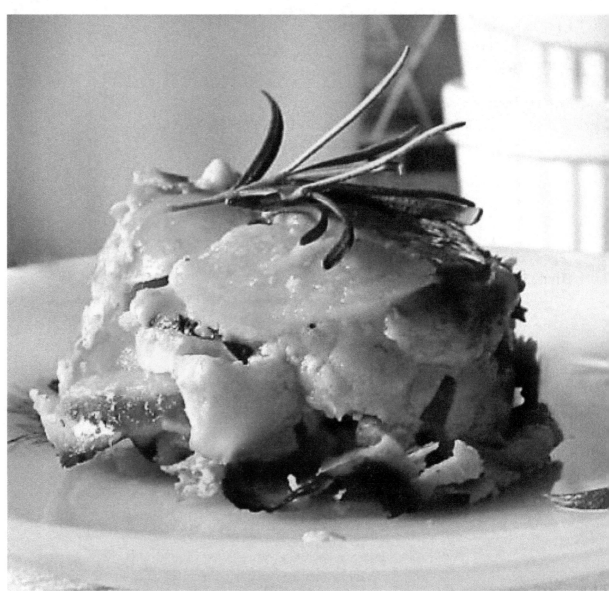

Preparation time: 10 minutes
Cooking time: 2 hours
Servings: 4

Ingredients:
- 1 pound cod fillets, cut into medium pieces
- 2 tablespoons parsley, chopped
- 4 ounces breadcrumbs
- 2 teaspoons lemon juice
- 2 eggs, whisked
- 2 ounces butter, melted
- ½ pint milk

- ½ pint shrimp sauce
- Salt and black pepper to the taste

Directions:
1. In a bowl, mix fish with crumbs, lemon juice, parsley, salt and pepper and stir.
2. Add butter to your Slow cooker, add milk and whisk well.
3. Add egg and fish mix, stir, cover and cook on High for 2 hours.
4. Divide between plates and serve with shrimp sauce on top.

Nutrition: calories 231, fat 3, fiber 5, carbs 10, protein 5

Shrimp and Rice Mix

Preparation time: 5 minutes
Cooking time: 1 hour and 30 minutes
Servings: 2

Ingredients:
- 1 pound shrimp, peeled and deveined
- 1 cup chicken stock
- ½ cup wild rice
- ½ cup carrots, peeled and cubed
- 1 green bell pepper, cubed
- ½ teaspoon turmeric powder
- ½ teaspoon coriander, ground
- 1 tablespoon olive oil
- 1 red onion, chopped
- A pinch of salt and black pepper
- 1 tablespoon cilantro, chopped

Directions:
1. In your slow cooker, mix the stock with the rice, carrots and the other ingredients except the shrimp, toss, put the lid on and cook on High for 1 hour.
2. Add the shrimp, toss, put the lid back on and cook on High for 30 minutes.
3. Divide the mix between plates and serve.

Nutrition: calories 232, fat 9, fiber 2, carbs 6, protein 8

Jambalaya

Preparation time: 10 minutes
Cooking time: 4 hours and 30 minutes
Servings: 8

Ingredients:
- 1 pound chicken breast, chopped
- 1 pound shrimp, peeled and deveined
- 2 tablespoons extra virgin olive oil
- 1 pound sausage, chopped
- 2 cups onions, chopped
- 1 and ½ cups rice
- 2 tablespoons garlic, chopped
- 2 cups green, yellow and red bell peppers, chopped
- 3 and ½ cups chicken stock
- 1 tablespoon Creole seasoning
- 1 tablespoon Worcestershire sauce
- 1 cup tomatoes, crushed

Directions:
1. Add the oil to your Slow cooker and spread.
2. Add chicken, sausage, onion, rice, garlic, mixed bell peppers, stock, seasoning, tomatoes and Worcestershire sauce, cover and cook on High for 4 hours.
3. Add shrimp, cover, cook on High for 30 minutes more, divide everything between plates and serve.

Nutrition: calories 251, fat 10, fiber 3, carbs 20, protein 25

Shrimp and Red Chard

Preparation time: 5 minutes
Cooking time: 1 hour
Servings: 2

Ingredients:
- 1 pound shrimp, peeled and deveined
- Juice of 1 lime
- 1 cup red chard, torn
- ½ cup tomato sauce
- 2 garlic cloves, minced
- 1 red onion, sliced
- 1 tablespoon olive oil
- ½ teaspoon sweet paprika
- A pinch of salt and black pepper
- 1 tablespoon parsley, chopped

Directions:
1. In your slow cooker, mix the shrimp with the lime juice, chard and the other ingredients, toss, put the lid on and cook on High for 1 hour.
2. Divide the mix into bowls and serve.

Nutrition: calories 200, fat 13, fiber 3, carbs 6, protein 11

Mushroom Tuna Mix

Preparation time: 5 minutes
Cooking time: 2 hours
Servings: 4

Ingredients:
- 14 ounces canned tuna, drained
- 16 ounces egg noodles
- 28 ounces cream of mushroom
- 1 cup peas, frozen
- 3 cups water
- 4 ounces cheddar cheese, grated
- ¼ cup breadcrumbs

Directions:
1. Add pasta and water to your Slow cooker, also add tuna, peas and cream, stir, cover and cook on High for 1 hour.
2. Add cheese, stir, spread breadcrumbs all over, cover, cook on High for 1 more hour, divide into bowls and serve.

Nutrition: calories 251, fat 6, fiber 1, carbs 20, protein 12

Chives Mussels

Preparation time: 5 minutes
Cooking time: 1 hour
Servings: 2

Ingredients:
- 1 pound mussels, debearded
- ½ teaspoon coriander, ground
- ½ teaspoon rosemary, dried
- 1 tablespoon lime zest, grated
- Juice of 1 lime
- 1 cup tomato passata
- ¼ cup chicken stock
- A pinch of salt and black pepper
- 1 tablespoon chives, chopped

Directions:
1. In your slow cooker, mix the mussels with the coriander, rosemary and the other ingredients, toss, put the lid on and cook on High for 1 hour.
2. Divide the mix into bowls and serve.

Nutrition: calories 200, fat 12, fiber 2, carbs 6, protein 9

Chili Mackerel

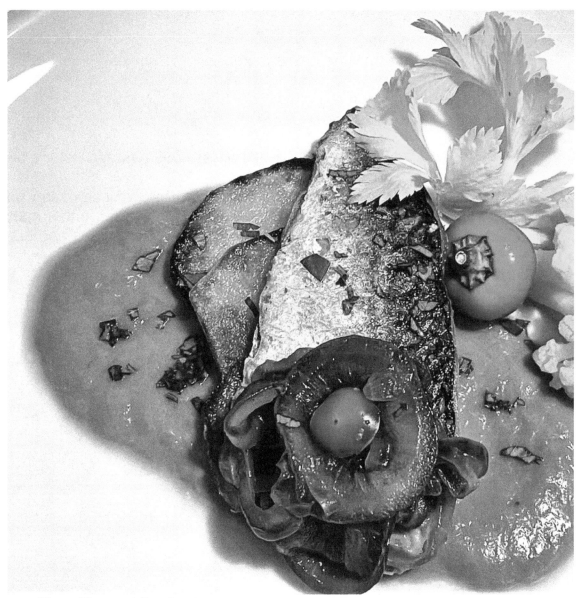

Preparation time: 10 minutes
Cooking time: 2 hours
Servings: 4

Ingredients:
- 18 ounces mackerel, cut into pieces
- 3 garlic cloves, minced
- 8 shallots, chopped
- 1 teaspoon dried shrimp powder
- 1 teaspoon turmeric powder
- 1 tablespoon chili paste

- 2 lemongrass sticks, cut into halves
- 1 small piece of ginger, chopped
- 6 stalks laska leaves
- 3 and ½ ounces water
- 5 tablespoons vegetable oil
- 1 tablespoon tamarind paste mixed with 3 ounces water
- Salt to the taste
- 1 tablespoon sugar

Directions:
1. In your blender, mix garlic with shallots, chili paste, turmeric powder and shrimp powder and blend well.
2. Add the oil to your Slow cooker, also add fish, spices paste, ginger, lemongrass, laska leaves, tamarind mix, water, salt and sugar, stir, cover, cook on High for 2 hours, divide between plates and serve.

Nutrition: calories 200, fat 3, fiber 1, carbs 20, protein 22

Calamari and Sauce

Preparation time: 10 minutes
Cooking time: 2 hours
Servings: 2

Ingredients:
- 1 pound calamari rings
- 2 scallions, chopped
- 2 garlic cloves, minced
- ½ cup heavy cream
- ½ cup chicken stock
- 1 tablespoon lime juice
- ½ cup black olives, pitted and halved
- A pinch of salt and black pepper
- 2 tablespoons chives, chopped

Directions:
1. In your slow cooker, mix the calamari with the scallions, garlic and the other ingredients except the cream, toss, put the lid on and cook on High for 1 hour.
2. Add the cream, toss, cook on High for 1 more hour, divide into bowls and serve.

Nutrition: calories 200, fat 12, fiber 2, carbs 5, protein 6

Chinese Mackerel

Preparation time: 10 minutes
Cooking time: 2 hours
Servings: 4

Ingredients:
- 2 pounds mackerel, cut into medium pieces
- 1 cup water
- 1 garlic clove, crushed
- 1 shallot, sliced
- 1-inch ginger piece, chopped
- 1/3 cup sake
- 1/3 cup mirin
- ¼ cup miso
- 1 sweet onion, thinly sliced
- 2 celery stalks, sliced
- 1 tablespoon rice vinegar
- 1 teaspoon Japanese hot mustard
- Salt to the taste
- 1 teaspoon sugar

Directions:
1. In your Slow cooker, mix mirin, sake, ginger, garlic and shallot.
2. Add miso, water and mackerel, stir, cover the slow cooker and cook on High for 2 hours.
3. Put onion and celery in a bowl and cover with ice water.
4. In another bowl, mix vinegar with salt, sugar and mustard and stir well.
5. Divide mackerel on plates, drain onion and celery well, mix with mustard dressing, divide next to mackerel and serve.

Nutrition: calories 300, fat 12, fiber 1, carbs 14, protein 20

Salmon Salad

Preparation time: 5 minutes
Cooking time: 3 hours
Servings: 2

Ingredients:
- 1 pound salmon fillets, boneless and cubed
- ¼ cup chicken stock
- 1 zucchini, cut with a spiralizer
- 1 carrot, sliced
- 1 eggplant, cubed
- ½ cup cherry tomatoes, halved
- 1 red onion, sliced
- ½ teaspoon turmeric powder
- ½ teaspoon chili powder
- ½ tablespoon rosemary, chopped
- A pinch of salt and black pepper
- 1 tablespoon chives, chopped

Directions:
1. In your slow cooker, mix the salmon with the zucchini, stock, carrot and the other ingredients,, toss , put the lid on and cook on High for 3 hours.
2. Divide the mix into bowls and serve.

Nutrition: calories 424, fat 15.1, fiber 12.4, carbs 28.1, protein 49

Mackerel and Lemon

Preparation time: 10 minutes
Cooking time: 2 hours
Servings: 4

Ingredients:
- 4 mackerels
- 3 ounces breadcrumbs
- Juice and rind of 1 lemon
- 1 tablespoon chives, finely chopped
- Salt and black pepper to the taste
- 1 egg, whisked
- 1 tablespoon butter
- 1 tablespoon vegetable oil
- 3 lemon wedges

Directions:
1. In a bowl, mix breadcrumbs with lemon juice, lemon rind, salt, pepper, egg and chives, stir very well and coat mackerel with this mix.
2. Add the oil and the butter to your Slow cooker and arrange mackerel inside.
3. Cover, cook on High for 2 hours, divide fish between plates and serve with lemon wedges on the side.

Nutrition: calories 200, fat 3, fiber 1, carbs 3, protein 12

Walnut Tuna Mix

Preparation time: 10 minutes
Cooking time: 3 hours
Servings: 2

Ingredients:
- 1 pound tuna fillets, boneless
- ½ tablespoon walnuts, chopped
- ½ cup chicken stock
- ½ teaspoon chili powder
- ½ teaspoon sweet paprika
- 1 red onion, sliced
- 2 tablespoons parsley, chopped
- A pinch of salt and black pepper

Directions:
1. In your slow cooker, mix the tuna with the walnuts, stock and the other ingredients, toss, put the lid on and cook on High for 3 hours.
2. Divide everything between plates and serve.

Nutrition: calories 200, fat 10, fiber 2, carbs 5, protein 9

Mussels and Sausage Mix

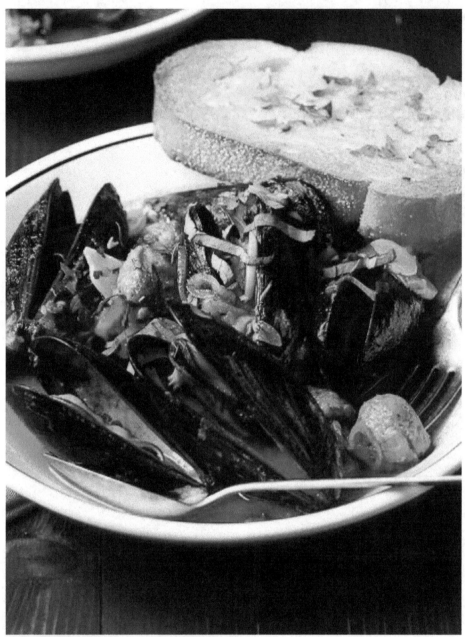

Preparation time: 5 minutes
Cooking time: 2 hours
Servings: 4

Ingredients:
- 2 pounds mussels, scrubbed and debearded
- 12 ounces amber beer
- 1 tablespoon olive oil
- 1 yellow onion, chopped

- 8 ounces spicy sausage
- 1 tablespoon paprika

Directions:
1. Grease your Slow cooker with the oil, add onion, paprika, sausage, mussels and beer, cover and cook on High for 2 hours.
2. Discard unopened mussels, divide the rest between bowls and serve.

Nutrition: calories 124, fat 3, fiber 1, carbs 7, protein 12

Almond Shrimp and Cabbage

Preparation time: 5 minutes
Cooking time: 1 hour
Servings: 2

Ingredients:
- 1 pound shrimp, peeled and deveined
- 1 cup red cabbage, shredded
- 1 tablespoon almonds, chopped
- 1 cup cherry tomatoes, halved
- 1 tablespoon balsamic vinegar
- 2 tablespoons olive oil
- ½ cup tomato passata
- A pinch of salt and black pepper

Directions:
1. In your slow cooker, mix the shrimp with the cabbage, almonds and the other ingredients, toss, put the lid on and cook on High for 1 hour.
2. Divide everything into bowls and serve.

Nutrition: calories 200, fat 13, fiber 3, carbs 6, protein 11

Conclusion
Did you indulge in attempting these brand-new and delicious recipes? unfortunately we have come to the end of this sluggish stove cookbook, I really desire it has really been to your liking. to boost your wellness and also health we would love to recommend you to integrate exercise and likewise a dynamic means of living in addition to comply with these excellent recipes, so regarding emphasize the improvements. we will certainly be back soon with other dramatically appealing vegan dishes, a huge hug, see you quickly.

CPSIA information can be obtained
at www.ICGtesting.com
Printed in the USA
LVHW060902290521
688445LV00038B/978